THE TRUE DEFINITION OF

BEAUTY

Facial Cosmetic Treatment's
Transformational Role in Modern
Beauty and Communication

DEDICATION

This book is dedicated to my mentors, patients, family, and friends. You have all taught me and inspired me to become a better doctor.

As doctors, we are able to achieve what we can today because of the work done by the giants of our field in the past. I consider myself fortunate to be able to stand on the shoulders of many great physicians and surgeons to further advance our field and help our patients.

TABLE OF CONTENTS

INTRODUCTION

The search for and appreciation of "beauty" is as old as time itself. As far back as we look in human history, we find the search for the beautiful. While certain perceptions of popular beauty may come and go, true beauty is timeless, and we all know it the instant we see it.

We may believe beauty is a subjective determination that's purely "in the eyes of the beholder," but while we each have different likes and dislikes, we also have a natural, hard-wired, and objective affinity towards certain aspects of a person's appearance. Understanding these underlying aspects allows us to see that the people we find attractive typically have the same features in common.

Studies have revealed that there is a mathematical basis for the facial ratios to which we are naturally attracted. Achieving these facial ratios is what creates a balanced and recognizably "attractive" face—and having this naturally balanced appearance can significantly improve one's confidence and ability to communicate with the world. In contrast, when time or life circumstances cause our natural features to become out of balance, it negatively impacts the way the world perceives us—and the way we perceive ourselves.

In our society's never-ending quest for beauty, we have often gotten it all wrong. The media loves to hold up a certain ideal which changes constantly and which is very rarely in line with the true definition of beauty. Rather than learning to appreciate our own unique beauty, we are prompted to become a mirror image of whatever celebrity is this season's "it" girl (or guy). Many cosmetic surgeons are more than happy to comply with this desire, resulting in the exaggerated and disproportionate appearances that have given cosmetic procedures a bad name.

It's no wonder we find ourselves confused by what true facial beauty is and how to achieve it.

This book is designed to answer the question: What is the true definition of beauty? (Or "handsomeness" in the case of men, which we'll include for our purposes in the use of the word "beauty" throughout this book.) It explores the ways in which people perceive beauty, as well as how men and women today are achieving their unique, balanced, ideal facial appearances, enabling them to communicate more effectively and in turn to live fuller lives.

In this book, we'll be covering:

- The science behind what we find beautiful and its implications for interpersonal communication

- How harnessing the power of one's appearance and nonverbal cues can drastically change a person's life

- How cosmetic surgery and cosmetic procedures have gotten a bad rap due to misconceptions and mistreatments

- How applying the "Golden Ratio" when performing cosmetic treatments can achieve powerful yet natural results

- How real-life, everyday people have enhanced their natural appearances (and their lives) through cosmetic treatment

- How to determine whether your cosmetic surgeon or laser eyelid and facial plastic surgeon is the right fit to achieve the results you want

It is my hope that this book will encourage you to look at beauty — true beauty — from a new perspective and will show you how modern advances in cosmetic procedures can enable individuals to dramatically improve their lives by restoring and reclaiming their natural, balanced appearances.

01

The Science Behind
What We Find
Beautiful (And What
It Means for
Communication)

Throughout history, human beings have searched for beauty and have revered it when they've found it. It's something we do without thinking. Back in Ancient Greece, when Aristotle was asked why people desire physical beauty, the great sage replied, "No one who is not blind could ask that question."

But why is this true? Why does beauty have such a hold over us—and how do our brains recognize it? Is it, as they say, "in the eyes of the beholder," or is there an objective measure of what we consider beautiful?

While it may surprise you, there is an objective measure—and the math to back it up. Regardless of personal preferences, we are all genetically hard-wired to find certain things beautiful. True beauty has a natural harmony to it, and this harmony sends signals that let our unconscious minds know we're in the presence of something beautiful.

IS THERE AN OBJECTIVE MEASURE OF WHAT WE CONSIDER BEAUTIFUL? (YES)

It all comes down to a mathematical ratio known as the "Golden Ratio." Developed by a mathematician in the 1200s by the name of Leonard Fibonacci, this ratio holds the key to the visual balance and harmony we unconsciously perceive in the things we find attractive.

Simply put (I promise this won't be a complicated math lesson!), Fibonacci introduced a series of numbers to Western European mathematics that had previously been studied in Indian mathematics. This series of numbers was:

1 1 2 3 5 8

This ratio holds the key to the visual balance and harmony

13 21 34

55 89

144...

$$1 + 1 = 2 \qquad 2 + 1 = 3 \qquad 2 + 3 = 5$$

$$3 + 5 = 8 \qquad \ldots \qquad \text{and so on.}$$

Figure 1: This ratio will always come out to 1:1.618

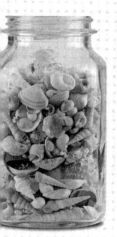

This sequence evolves by taking the first number and adding it to the following number to generate the next number in the sequence.

When you take any two successive numbers from the Fibonacci Sequence (in other words, any numbers that directly follow one another) and determine their ratio, this ratio will always come out to 1:1.618, or what is known as the "Golden Ratio."

Why the "Golden Ratio"? Because this incredible ratio can be found in countless instances in nature. From the branching of trees to the arrangement of leaves on a stem, the Golden Ratio pops up again and again.

Let's take a look at some examples.

etc.

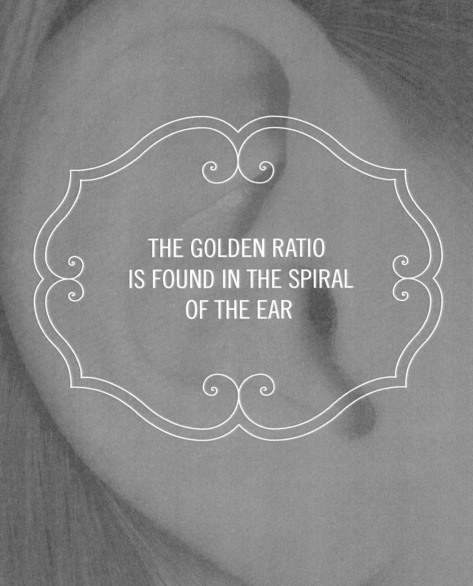

THE GOLDEN RATIO
IS FOUND IN THE SPIRAL
OF THE EAR

THE GOLDEN RATIO IN ACTION

The first embodiment of the Golden Ratio is a spiral shape.

When you create squares that are the width of each number in the Fibonacci sequence, you get a diagram that looks like Figure 2.

If you look from the outside in, the numbers in each box follow the Fibonacci sequence (1 plus 2 equals 3, 2 plus 3 equals 5, 3 plus 5 equals 8 and so on). When we connect these boxes from the inside of the diagram out, they create a spiral pattern, as illustrated by the teal line.

We see this spiral in many instances in nature, from the shape of a seashell…

…to the structure of the human ear.

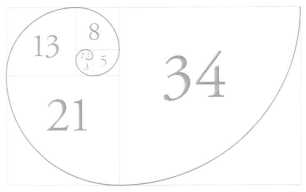

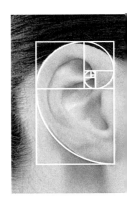

Figure 2: We see this spiral in many instances in nature

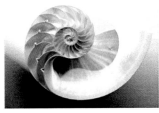

When we remove the spiral line from the diagram, the Golden Ratio creates a rectangle that looks like Figure 3.

Once again, each block in the sequence adds to the next to create the following number, in accordance with the ratio of 1:1.618. The lengths of the lines between these squares are all in keeping with the Golden Ratio.

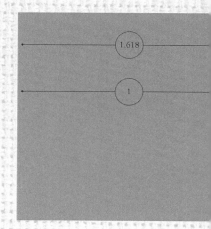

1:1.618

During the Renaissance, many artists worked with the lines of this Golden Ratio in mind. Architects constructed buildings like Notre Dame Cathedral that contained the ratios of 1:1.618 in their design.

Lines of these ratios can also be found in Leonardo da Vinci's famous paintings *Mona Lisa* and *The Last Supper*.

These are just a few of the countless examples you can find of the Golden Ratio, both in the beauty of nature and in the pieces of artwork we hold up as beautiful. The Golden Ratio is everywhere, and it provides us with the mathematical key to true, natural beauty.

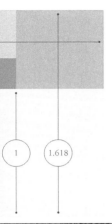

Figure 3: The
Golden Ratio
provides us with
the mathematical
key to true,
natural beauty

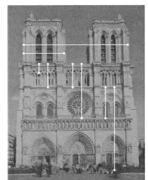

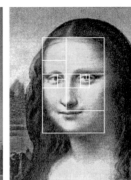

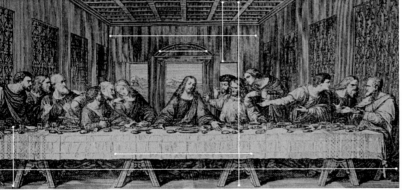

WHAT THIS MEANS FOR HUMAN RELATIONS

Unless they're drawn out for us, as in the examples below, our perception of the Golden Ratio occurs on a subconscious level. Regardless of ethnic background, current fads or personal preference, the more a person's face contains balance in harmony with the Golden Ratio, the more attractive we perceive that person to be.[1] See Figure 4.

This has much deeper implications than simply judging who is the "fairest of them all." The way the world perceives us greatly impacts the way the world relates to us (and, in turn, the way we view ourselves).

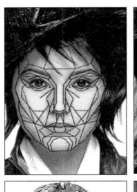
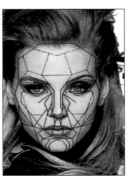
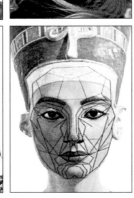

Figure 4: The Golden Ratio occurs on a subconscious level

02

Harnessing the Power of Appearance in Non-Verbal Communication

Our face is our calling card, and when its various aspects are out of balance, it can have a significant impact on the quality of our relationships and our lives.

First impressions are formed within the first seven seconds of meeting someone.[2] As much as we'd like to consider ourselves evolved and egalitarian, and as much as we may strive to treat each person equally, the scientific truth is that our brains are hard-wired to deduce certain things from someone's appearance. We may not even realize we're doing it, but we do, to a large extent, "judge a book by its cover." We can't help it.

Consider this: Researchers estimate that only 7% of our words come across in conversation, while 38% of our vocal tone and 55% of non-verbal communication is perceived.[3]

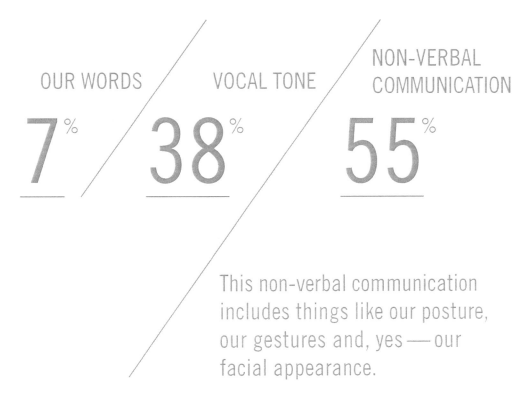

OUR WORDS   VOCAL TONE   NON-VERBAL COMMUNICATION

7%   38%   55%

This non-verbal communication includes things like our posture, our gestures and, yes — our facial appearance.

When we communicate, our words don't speak for us nearly as loudly as these other factors do. This is why our communication and relationships with others can be so greatly improved by making sure our face is communicating what we want it to — that our "calling card" is an accurate representation of who we really are and how we really feel.

DOES AN IMPROVED APPEARANCE GIVE YOU AN ADVANTAGE?

In a word—yes.

In her book, *Survival of the Prettiest*,[4] Nancy Etcoff observed the ways in which we routinely evaluate the attractiveness of one another. She argued that our sensitivity to beauty is a biological adaptation that was shaped by natural selection.

Etcoff noted that babies stare significantly longer at the faces of adults who are appealing, and that mothers of "attractive babies" display more intense bonding behaviors towards their children. She also observed that we often try to please people we find attractive, with no expectation of immediate reward or reciprocal gestures. I don't think it's a scientific breakthrough to suggest that in everyday life, attractive adults are more likely to "get away" with things—whether it's little infractions like cheating on examinations or larger offenses like shoplifting.

We often try to please people we find attractive

Our appearance plays a key role in the non-verbal communication we send out into the world and, in turn, influences the way the world relates to us.

Whether you'd like to gain the respect of your col-
leagues, make friends more easily or just communicate with your loved ones better, your appearance
either helps or hinders you.

Want further evidence that our appearances affect
the way we're perceived? Take a look at Figure 5 and
consider which one you'd consider "masculine" and
which "feminine."

Figure 5: The degree of
facial contrasts contribute
to the relative masculinity
or femininity of a face

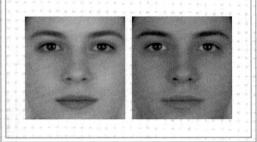

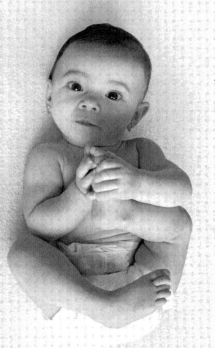

What did you decide? Did you say
the left appeared more feminine and the
right more masculine? These were the
findings of many people who took this
test. In actuality, this is a photo of the
same person with different color contrasts
in the eyes and mouth region in the
two photos.

These photos were from a scientific study by Harvard psychologist Richard Russell, who studied the differences in the facial contrast between men and women.[5] He lightened the eyes and lips in the right photo and darkened the eyes and lips in the left photo. The results of the test proved his point that the degree of facial contrasts contribute to the relative masculinity or femininity of a face.

It turns out that, in general, men have fewer differences in the contrast in their faces. To say it another way, men have less color differentiation across the different parts of their faces. On the other hand, women have extensive differentiation in contrast in their faces (or more differences in the color in different parts of their faces). This is especially true in the eye and mouth regions. Women's lips also have more natural color as compared to men.

As women intuitively know, people look at the mouth and eye area first when viewing another person.

These are the two most powerful areas of the face for non-verbal communication with the outside world. This is why women highlight their eyes by wearing mascara and eye shadow and their lips by wearing lip liner and lipstick. By adding color to these areas, their faces are perceived by others as being more feminine.

Take a look at these photos of the same woman (Figure 6). In one she is wearing makeup and in the other she is not. Which photo appears more feminine to you? Which is more attractive?

I'm willing to guess that you chose the photo on the right. Thanks to makeup, the increased color of the woman's eyes and lips stimulate the non-verbal messages sent to our unconscious brains that assess beauty and feminine attractiveness. This is an example of how our subconscious brain's hardwiring causes us to find certain facial features and ratios beautiful.

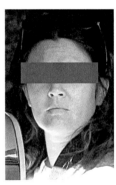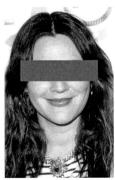

Figure 6: This is an example of how our subconscious brain's hardwiring causes us to find certain facial features and ratios beautiful

WHAT YOUR FACE SAYS ABOUT YOU

There are two parts of the face that are perceived most strongly in communication. The first is the area around the eyes and the second is the area around the mouth. When we first see one another, our brains quickly scan these two areas for non-verbal cues. Irregularities in these areas affect our assessment of a person.

Optimizing these areas can pay big dividends in the way that other people perceive us. This can be accomplished by doing something as simple as using makeup to highlight certain areas and smooth out others, or wearing flattering glasses to bring attention to the eyes.

Unfortunately, sometimes as we age makeup and glasses aren't enough. As we get older our faces can begin to send more and more non-verbal messages that are inconsistent with the way we truly feel.

Specifically, consider the eyes. As we age our eyelids can begin to droop and look heavy.

This may be due to a lower eyelid height, heaviness of the upper or lower eyelid or an eyebrow falling into the upper eyelid space. Whatever the cause, having baggy, puffy eyes can make a person look tired, sleepy, old or sick. It's been said that the eyes are the windows to the soul, yet when our eyes are projecting an image that isn't us—when people start commenting on how tired we look when in fact we feel fine—we can start to feel like we truly embody the message we see in the mirror. We begin to feel old or sick or tired because we always look as if we are.

EYES

People look at the
mouth and eye area
first when viewing
another person

+

MOUTH

Rejuvenating your eyes
can have an incredible
impact on the way you
feel about yourself
and the way the world
interacts with you.

HOW PUTTING YOUR BEST FACE FORWARD CAN IMPROVE COMMUNICATION (AND YOUR LIFE)

When you enhance your natural beauty, it enables you
to communicate more effectively with people across all
areas of your life.

By making natural-looking changes in your appearance that allow others to better relate to you, you gain a competitive edge in your business interactions and improve communication with friends and loved ones. The non-verbal cues you send out are more in line with who you really are and how you really feel.

Working with a cosmetic surgeon who takes the time to assess your face on an individual basis and who has the experience and specialization to customize the right procedures for your needs makes all the difference in the world. It results in an enhanced natural beauty that directly impacts communication in a positive, and often life-changing, way.

The proper cosmetic procedures — performed by a surgeon who understands true, balanced beauty and can bring out the unique beauty in each of his patients — can be transformative. I am able to take patients from a place of disconnect and unhappiness to a more harmonious and positive life experience, and it never ceases to be rewarding to me.

Unfortunately, many people are hesitant at the thought of having any sort of cosmetic procedure or surgery. In the next two chapters we'll explore the ways that cosmetic procedures have gotten a bad rap and then learn what the proper approach to cosmetic procedures should be.

When you enhance your natural beauty, it enables you to communicate more effectively

03

How We've Gotten It Wrong: Why Cosmetic Procedures Have a Bad Rap

From the overly puffy lips of celebrity debutants to obvious and unnatural face lifts on aging actresses, the media has shown us plenty of examples of why cosmetic procedures have gotten a bad name.

When performed responsibly, cosmetic surgery and cosmetic procedures can offer patients so much value. Yet they've gotten a bad connotation for a reason. While we know the media tends to focus on the negative aspects of any given topic, pitfalls in the cosmetic surgery industry do exist, and it's important that patients are aware of these pitfalls so that they can choose a cosmetic surgeon who will give them the positive results they're seeking.

Let's take a look at the problems with cosmetic procedures that have led people to view them negatively.

LACK OF SPECIALIZATION

In the past, there were general surgeons who were able to perform almost any procedure. But today's sophisticated medicine has evolved into so many facets that any doctor performing a procedure must be well-trained in that specific area. A "jack of all trades" won't cut it anymore.

Unfortunately, as more and more people enter the field of cosmetic and eyelid procedures, many practicing surgeons just don't have the qualifications and experience necessary to expertly perform certain procedures.

A "jack of all trades" won't cut it anymore

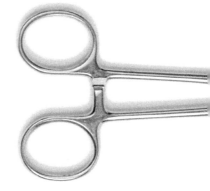

Patients who don't realize this don't take the time to properly investigate their surgeon. This can lead to results that are — in a good scenario — less than perfect.

Bringing forth a person's natural beauty requires a specialized and sophisticated approach that not all cosmetic surgeons take.

A surgeon that doesn't specialize cannot effectively perform work in certain areas. Everyone tries to do well and produce good results, of course, but if you don't have the training and experience necessary then the results you produce will be less than optimal (to put it kindly). This is why I focus specifically on the face, with a specialization around the eyes. By continuing to hone my skills and keeping up-to-date with medical breakthroughs, as well as through my experience performing thousands of successful procedures, I am able to give my patients the quality results that they deserve.

For instance, let's consider the issues that can arise with the improper use of under-eye fillers (Figure 7).

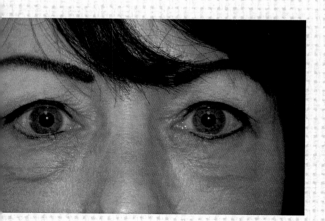

Figure 7: If you don't have the training and experience necessary, the results you produce will be less than optimal (to put it kindly)

One of the most common causes of dark circles under the eyes is fullness due to fat changes that occur in and around the eyes as we age. The advent of facial fillers such as Juvederm,® Restylane,® Belotero,® Radiesse,® Bellafill,® Fat, Silicone, and Sculptra® has proven very useful in reversing age-related volume loss in the face.

Many doctors also use these fillers to camouflage the appearance of dark circles under the eyes (also due to a lack of fat, which causes a sunken appearance to the under-eye area). I myself have used fillers in this region to address this specific cause of dark circles under the eyes.

As we age, the fat around our eyes can shift forward into the lower eyelid region as a result of the relaxation of retaining ligaments and sheets in this area. I have seen many problems arise from people having fillers put under their eyes to camouflage these fat changes.

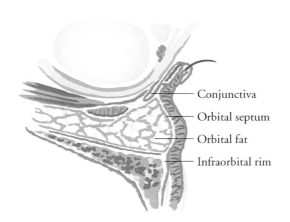

Figure 8: As we age, the fat around our eyes can shift forward into the lower eyelid region

Conjunctiva

Orbital septum

Orbital fat

Infraorbital rim

You can also see this in the sets of photos here:

Figure 9: The
more effective
procedure is
surgery around
the eyes

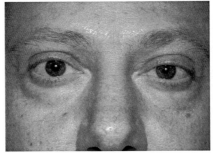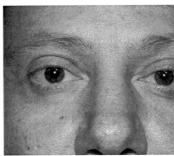

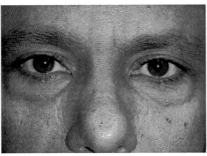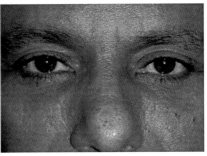

Figure 10: This requires
thorough, expert knowledge
of the eye region

This "bags under the eyes" effect can be further accentuated by loss of volume in the cheek region.

Today, certain practitioners are injecting fillers under the eyes to camouflage the fat pushing forward in this region. While expert injectors with great experience can be successful in improving the appearance of bulging fat in this area, the more effective procedure is surgery around the eyes to remove and, in some cases, reposition the fat. This requires thorough, expert knowledge of the eye region, which many practitioners lack.

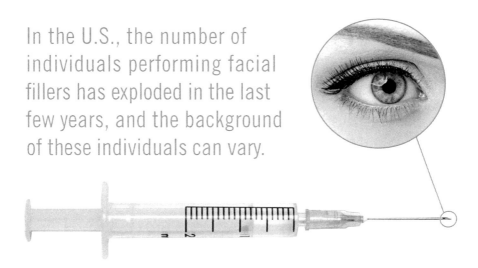

In the U.S., the number of individuals performing facial fillers has exploded in the last few years, and the background of these individuals can vary.

Traditional cosmetic specialists such as oculoplastic surgeons, facial plastic surgeons, oral maxillofacial plastic surgeons, general plastic surgeons, and cosmetic dermatologists are all using these fillers.

Unfortunately, doctors with less-extensive facial background, including dentists, general surgeons, family medicine doctors, internal medical doctors, pediatricians, emergency room physicians, allergists, and gynecologists are also using facial fillers.

Finally, non-physician extenders such as physician assistants, nurse practitioners, general nurses, and medical estheticians can also be involved with injecting fillers in the face. These individuals can have limited medical background, depending on the state in which they are operating.

The age-related changes around the eyes dramatically affect the way others perceive us, so it's understandable that so many people are seeking out ways to improve their appearance in this area. What's scary is that these people often end up in the hands of the diverse—and not always qualified—group of facial filler injectors described above.

FILLERS

Many of these injectors don't perform any facial surgery, so they use what knowledge they have, but this often works to the disadvantage of the patients. People without knowledge of facial anatomy can create irregular results when using facial fillers in general, and in the eyelid region specifically. You can see one such result in Figure 11.

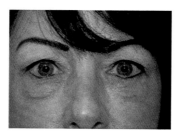

Figure 11: Fillers placed under the eyes often create irregular contours

I have no doubt that many of these practitioners have nothing but the best intentions when performing facial filler injections, but they don't have the expertise necessary to truly help their patients.

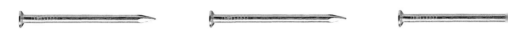

The large majority of injectors out there are likely to cause irregularities

It's been said that when all you've mastered is a hammer, everything looks like a nail. Expert facial rejuvenation requires a broad base of knowledge, as well as skill in using a large variety of facial rejuvenation tools and techniques. The large number of new injectors, who come from varying backgrounds and who have various skills, means that not all who are providing injections have what it takes. Injecting the lower lids should only be performed by those with advanced knowledge and experience in this area. The large majority of injectors with insufficient knowledge and skill are likely to cause irregularities in the lower lid area, and may actually make patients' appearances worse than they were before they sought help.

The second issue that arises involves the material used in these injections. Certain fillers, called hyaluronic acids (Juvederm®, Restylane®, Belotero®), are able to be dissolved by injecting a product called a hyaluronidase into them. This enzyme can be used to dissolve any of the hyaluronic acid products that are injected into the face and is only available commercially to doctors. This dissolution can be necessary when the filler affects the blood supply in a part of the face. It can also be useful to correct problems when these fillers lead to bad results.

I have frequently used these hyaluronidases to dissolve fillers that were badly placed in patients. Note the irregular-looking filler in the lower eyelid region of the woman in Figure 12, and how this region looked after dissolving the filler with hyaluronidase:

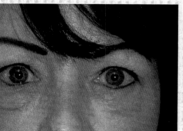 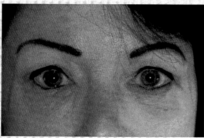

Figure 12: Note the irregular-looking filler in the lower eyelid region

Recently, I've been dissolving more and more badly-placed filler for patients from around the world who come to see me for my eyelid rejuvenation techniques. I am happy that I have a product that works against the major class of fillers injected into this region (hyaluronic acids). Since it can dissolve this material, I am able to help these patients.

Unfortunately, the other classes of fillers used (Radiesse,® Silicone, Sculptra,® Bellafill) don't have anything available to dissolve them. As a result, errors made with these fillers are very difficult to reverse. I can sometimes use invasive surgical techniques to remove these products, but often there is nothing that can be done to help these patients. It is my strong recommendation that these types of permanent and partially permanent filler products not be placed in the eyelid region.

Although facial fillers have been a great tool in helping practitioners reverse age-related changes in their patients' faces, it's important for patients to know the background and experience of the people injecting them. Some plastic surgeons actually have their more qualified or experienced physician extenders do their filler work for them, so in those cases having the plastic surgeon inject those fillers could be a mistake. While some physician extenders have great background and experience, one should always be careful, because many do not.

In the end, when dealing with an expert, knowledge-able, and skilled injector, using fillers to help the eyelid region is an option. Still, most cases would be best served by having an expert in eyelid rejuvenation assess the situation. If indicated, consider a more definitive surgical option to correct the problem rather than trying to hide the problem with fillers.

I strongly encourage anyone considering cosmetic proce-dures to educate themselves and thoroughly investigate their doctors to ensure they have expertise in the specific area of work to be done. Otherwise they could face major disappointments that are often irreversible and can even be dangerous.

LACK OF FOCUS ON NATURAL RESULTS

Even doctors who specialize may take a flawed approach to their work. Patients often request (and doctors perform) a procedure with a nearsighted goal in mind. Rather than focusing on making the entire face look better, they zero in on one feature to the exclusion of everything else, causing results that look unnatural or heavy-handed. Think of some of the overly full lips and radically lifted eyes and cheekbones you've seen on people who have obviously "had work done." These kinds of drastic (and often unattractive) appearances are the result of not considering the face as a whole.

In my practice, I stress the importance of achieving total facial balance with every procedure I perform. By paying attention to the Golden Ratio regardless of the procedure, I'm able to optimize a patient's appearance by enhancing the natural beauty that is unique to each person. The results "fit" with their other features and make them look like an improved version of themselves, not a science experiment gone wrong.

A surgeon must have the intuition and authority to say no to a patient who requests an unnecessary procedure or who does not seem like a good candidate. In turn, patients must be educated to view cosmetic surgery and cosmetic procedures as a means of revealing their natural beauty, not of turning themselves into someone they are not.

YOU SHOULDN'T JUST FOCUS ON THE EXTERNAL

I know—that seems a tad obvious, doesn't it? The field of cosmetic surgery is all about the externals, right? After all, what we work on are people's appearances.

But there is so much more to a successful, life-changing procedure than just a focus on the external. It's this shallow "beauty for beauty's sake" focus that makes people want to look like their favorite celebrity, or to get procedures they don't need and to take procedures to unnatural extremes.

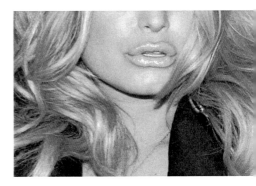

FOCUS

ON THE FACE AS A WHOLE

Figure 13: There is so much more to a successful, life-changing procedure than just a focus on the external

Truly qualified surgeons must be able to see all sides of a cosmetic procedure experience — the emotional, the mental and spiritual, as well as the physical — and they must be able to educate their patients on all of these aspects to make sure their patients fully understand the process they will be undergoing. Whatever procedure is being done should be an empowering experience that positively affects the patient, both inside and out.

AN EXAMPLE OF MISSING THE MARK

One procedure you see a lot of in Hollywood these days is cheek fillers. Actors seek out this procedure because full cheeks are associated with youthfulness, and as we all know, youth sells in Hollywood.

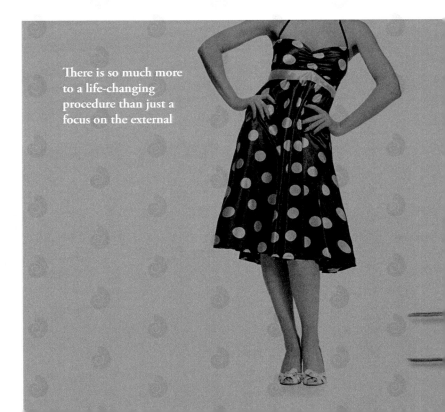

There is so much more to a life-changing procedure than just a focus on the external

Cheek fillers can be a good and effective enhancement when performed correctly. The problem arises when this area is treated by itself, without creating proper balance by addressing other parts of the face.

While the patients' cheeks may be fuller, if their jaw line or other neighboring areas are not re-volumized to provide balance, something just looks "off." One part of the face appears younger while the rest still looks old. Instances like this clearly show why a more comprehensive approach to cosmetic procedures is so important.

During the aging process, the face loses fat asymmetrically; some areas change more quickly than others. Facial re-volumization is necessary to create a balanced look so that one area of the face doesn't seem strange or out of place in relation to another.

Let's go back to our hard-wiring for a moment. Studies have shown that the human brain expects to see a smooth sweep or curve from temple to cheek to jaw line to chin. If there is a break in this curve, the brain tells us that a person is less vibrant and probably older.

Balancing out the whole face is the only way to ensure a harmonious and natural look that is appealing and attractive.

By being aware of these pitfalls in cosmetic surgery, patients can actively seek to avoid them. Be sure to check out Chapter 7 for some helpful things to keep in mind when considering which doctor to choose for your cosmetic procedure. There are doctors out there who give cosmetic procedures a good name, and you owe it to yourself to make sure you have found one.

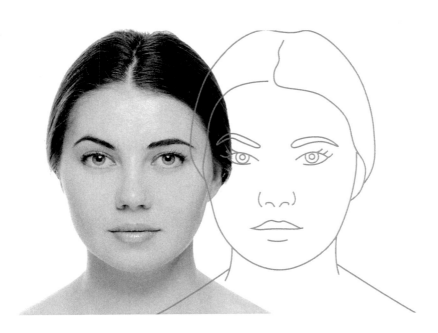

04

Applying the
Golden Ratio
to Achieve
Natural Beauty

The true definition of beauty isn't following the latest trend or seeking a certain cookie cutter look. Nearly any plastic surgeon can provide those kinds of results. Achieving optimal natural beauty requires an understanding of facial balance and how to enhance a person's appearance using the Golden Ratio we discussed in Chapter 1.

When I help a patient with his or her appearance, I pay very close attention to facial balance. I am careful to incorporate the principles of the Golden Ratio in order to create results that are powerful, yet natural. Referencing the Golden Ratio enables me to find the individual, naturally perfect ratios of each person's face and help make these ratios more visible to the world. I am seeking to reclaim the natural beauty which was always theirs to have, or to reveal the potential beauty that has been obstructed or changed by unbalanced features.

Let's take a look at an example of how the Golden Ratio can transform a person's appearance.

The woman in Figure 14 was upset because she kept receiving feedback that she seemed stern or unfriendly. If you take a look at her "before" picture on the left, then compare it to the "after" picture on the right, you can see that she seems more friendly and approachable in the second picture.

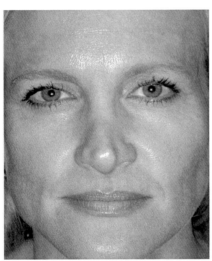 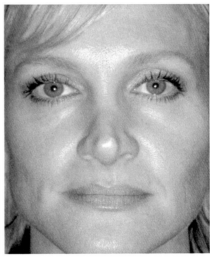

I was able to accomplish this change with one quick outpatient procedure that altered only one part of her face to restore a more balanced appearance.

Figure 14: She kept receiving feedback that she seemed stern or unfriendly

To see how I did this, take a look at the blue highlighted portion of the Fibonacci spiral below. Then compare this portion to the arc of the patient's eyebrow after her procedure. See Figure 15.

As you can see, after their restoration this woman's brows were higher and their arc more congruent with the arc of the Fibonacci spiral. The result was simple yet powerful, opening up her whole face while at the same time looking completely natural.

Truly successful cosmetic procedures keep the patient's natural facial ratios in mind. Whether I'm restoring an individual to a former version of themselves — when their face was more in balance — or working to reveal the potential beauty within, my focus is always on achieving balanced, natural results. These are the kinds of results that change lives (as you will see in the Chapter 6).

Figure 15: The result was simple yet powerful

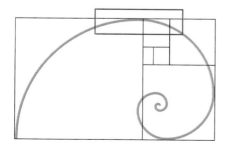

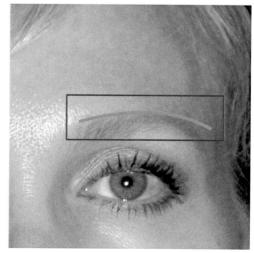

05

Rejuvenation vs.
Transformation

When it comes to helping patients Restore, Reveal and Reclaim™ their natural beauty, there are two specific ways this can be accomplished: by rejuvenation and by transformation.

D DETERIORATION

D DEFLATION

D DESCENT

REJUVENATION

Rejuvenation of a patient's natural beauty involves restoring their appearance to one they enjoyed in the past. For instance:

- Restoring the skin to the way it looked before being damaged by years of environmental factors such as sun exposure

- Restoring the eyelid or eyebrow region to the way it looked when a patient was younger

- Restoring a patient's overall appearance to a younger, fuller, and more symmetrical balance

Rejuvenation deals with reversing or undoing the effects of what I call the "3 D's of Aging":

THE 3 D'S OF AGING

1   Deterioration of the facial skin

2   Deflation of the face

3   Descent of the eyelids and face

Deterioration of the facial skin sometimes occurs naturally over the passage of time and as a normal result of aging, but I often see patients with premature aging and deterioration brought on by factors like smoking, stress, diet and — the biggest factor of them all — sun exposure. Sun exposure can drastically damage the skin and can be easily prevented with the daily use of a broad spectrum sun block. Other instances of facial deterioration include acne scars, age spots, and superficial pigmentation.

Figure 16: Before and after RESET Laser Skin Resurfacing

There are several ways to treat deterioration. Certain medications like Tretinoin and Hydroquinone can help repair the damage done to skin tissue. Cosmetic procedures can also reverse skin deterioration. Chemical peels, dermabrasion and laser skin resurfacing all help to restore the skin to an earlier, healthier state.

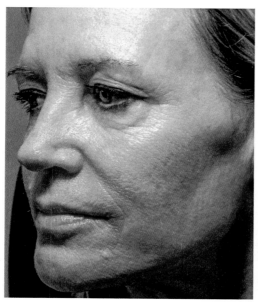 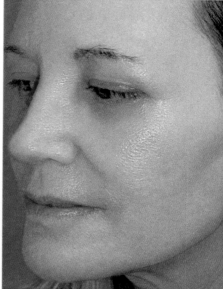

Figures 18–19: Before and after
RESET Laser Skin Resurfacing

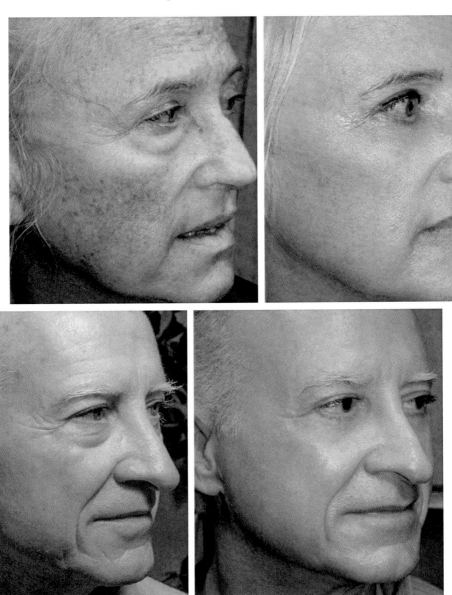

I prefer laser skin resurfacing, as it allows for a more customized approach based on each patient's specific needs. During this procedure, laser energy is applied to the patient's face in quick bursts. With the first pass of the laser beam, old skin is vaporized. Subsequent passes cause the collagen in the underlying layers to tighten, leaving smoother, healthier skin.

Another way to rejuvenate skin deterioration is with Broad Based Light™ (BBL™) treatments. Recent research performed at the Stanford University School of Medicine has shown that BBL™ treatments can cause both short-term and long-term improvement. In addition, the research shows that the device causes changes in the actual DNA of the skin cells that makes them behave like younger cells — not just causing an improvement in the appearance of skin, but actually changing the quality of the skin itself.

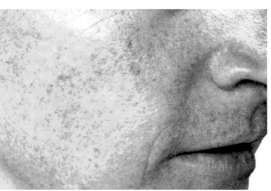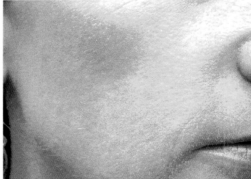

Figure 17: Before and After BBL

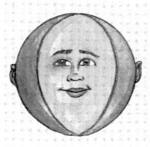

"Inflated Beach Ball"

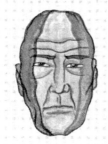

"Deflated Beach Ball"

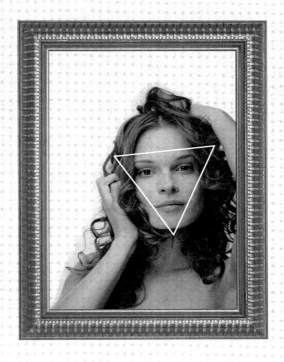

Figure 20: Deflation can best be described using the analogy of a beach ball

Deflation can best be described using the analogy of a beach ball. When we are young our faces are full and round—wider at the eyes and cheeks and narrower at the chin, much like an inverted triangle. As we age our faces start to "deflate," resulting in droopy, sagging skin, wrinkles and an overall narrower appearance. Picture a beach ball filled with air—round and full—and then picture that same beach ball as it begins to deflate. It becomes wrinkled and droopy, more of a sagging oval than a full, round circle.

Popular and effective treatments for deflation include the selective use of dermal fillers in my Radiant*Lift*® treatment. Radiant*Lift*® is an exciting new non-surgical face lift procedure in which a dermal filler is injected into specific fat-support regions. The facial skin itself is improved by reducing age spots and facial redness so that the skin appears more radiant. The re-volumizing portion of this procedure restores the three-dimensional structure to the soft tissue, filling and lifting the over-lying facial skin and restoring the face to its natural fullness. By improving the skin deterioration and facial deflation, as well as helping to camouflage facial descent (3 out of the 3 D's of Aging), this Radiant*Lift*® treatment creates synergistic results. It is a powerful rejuvenation procedure that occurs in a safe and comfortable office setting and has a quick recovery time.

Figure 21: Pre and post Radiant*Lift*®

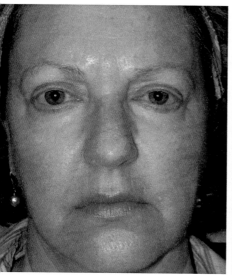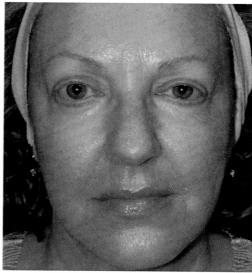

THE DEEPER MEANING BEHIND "BITCHY RESTING FACE"

Miscommunication can occur when heavy upper lids or baggy lower lids with Festoons or Malar Mounds make us appear tired, sick or older than we really are. It can also occur when our inner brow furrows and the corners of our mouth start to droop.

I once saw a video featuring a comedian speaking about her "Bitchy Resting Face." In it, she made fun of the fact that people are sensitive to each other's facial expressions, especially when the corners of the mouth droop, making us look "bitchy" to others. This condition isn't just a joke; in my practice patients have frequently expressed their dislike for their "Older Bitchy Face."

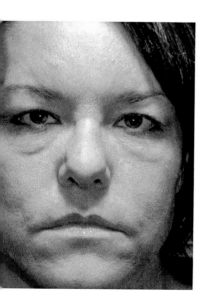

They are upset that they appear mad, angry or sad.

Figure 22: Patients have frequently expressed their dislike for their "Older Bitchy Face"

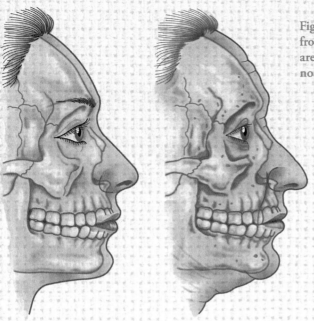

Figure 23: The folds we see from the nose to the mouth are actually a result of the nose falling into the face

Though it is true that downturned mouths can be seen in younger individuals, in the vast majority of cases they appear as people get older. Our faces age in a three-dimensional way, through changes in our bones, facial fat and skin layers. A downturned mouth is based in changes that occur in our teeth and jaws. With age the jaw starts to rotate backwards, and as it falls back into the deeper face, the skin around this area falls backwards as well.

In Figure 23, you can see the increase in the openness of the skeleton around the nose. The folds we see from the nose to the mouth (known as nasolabial folds) are actually a result of the nose falling into the face.

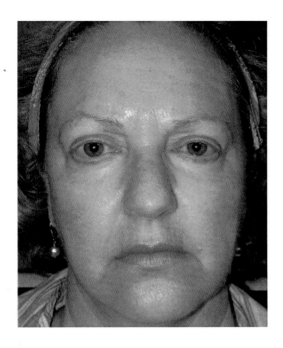

Figure 24: It is this folding inwards that causes the corner of the mouth to droop and makes us appear mad

In Figure 24, you can see the deeper bony changes that cause these folds (melolabial folds or "puppet lines") to develop from the corners of the mouth to the jaw line.

It is this folding inwards that causes the corner of the mouth to droop and makes us appear mad, sad and—for lack of a better word—"bitchy."

People who are frustrated with downturned corners around their mouth can also undergo a Radiant*Lift*® procedure. It is very effective in improving this condition and restoring a refreshed appearance to this part of the face that is so important for nonverbal communication.

Sometimes younger individuals have issues with down-turned corners of the mouth. For them, it is usually related to an over-action of the depressor anguli oris muscle. People who have an overactive depressor anguli oris muscle may want to reverse their "Bitchy Resting Face" with a small amount of BOTOX®. This is often an effective solution.

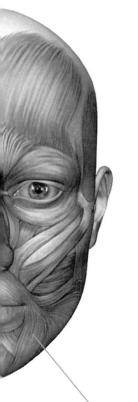

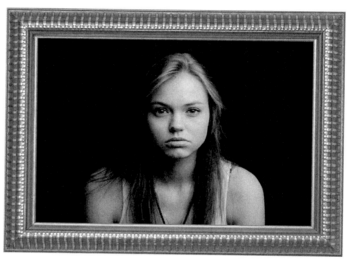

Figure 25: Sometimes younger individuals have issues with downturned corners of the mouth

DEPRESSOR
ANGULI ORIS

Descent of either the upper or lower eyelids is another common result of aging. It causes the eyes to look tired, sick and can cause a patient to look older than they really are. Drooping and sagging eyelids can even block a patient's upper vision in extreme cases. Descent can be seen in several conditions:

1 Drooping or heavy eyelids

2 Drooping eyebrows

3 Lower eyelid bags and/or "Festoons"

Drooping or Heavy Eyelids

Drooping or heavy eyelids can occur due to two separate conditions. Figure 26 shows a brow which descends into the eyelid space with age.

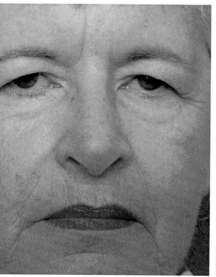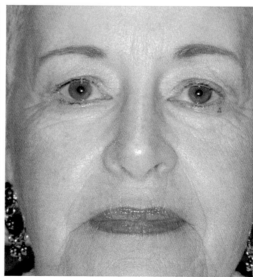

Figure 26: Pre and post browlift

Figure 27:
Redundant tissue
in the eyelid

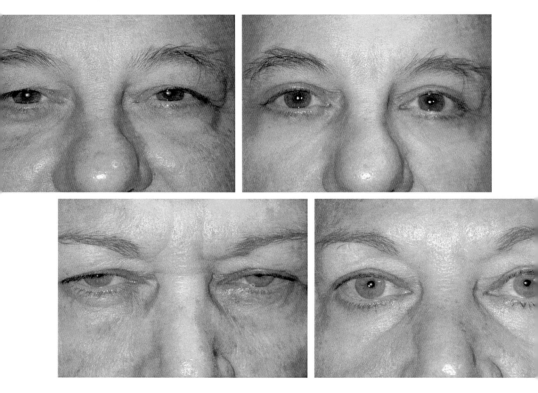

Figure 28: Pre and post
Levator Advancement
(Drooping Eyelid)

Figure 27 is an example of redundant tissue in the eyelid itself.

For drooping or heavy eyelids, shown in Figure 28, I can use eyelid surgery and eye lifts (or "levator advancement") to carefully isolate, adjust and raise the eyelids until they're at the proper height — all through a quick outpatient surgery.

Drooping Eyebrows

For patients with drooping eyebrows, fixing the eyelids alone won't fully open up the eyes. A procedure directly addressing the eyebrows is needed.

Although there are a number of ways to raise a drooping eyebrow, one of the best methods is the Minimal-Incision Brow Lift. The Minimal-Incision Brow Lift raises the drooping eyebrow to create a naturally awake look. The effect is not stiff or forced. As you can see from the photos below, patients look much more approachable and friendly after treatment in Figure 29.

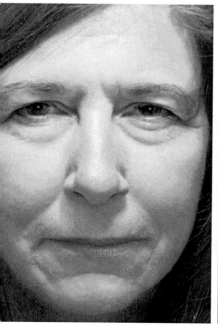
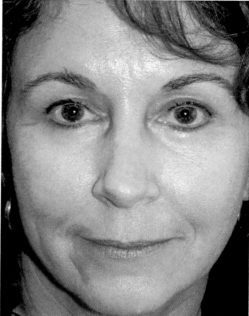

Figure 29: Before and After
Minimal Incision Browlift
and Lower Lid Rejuvenation

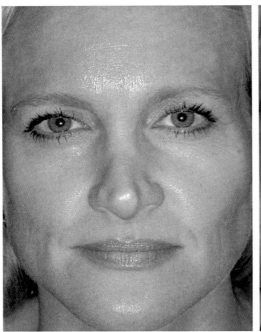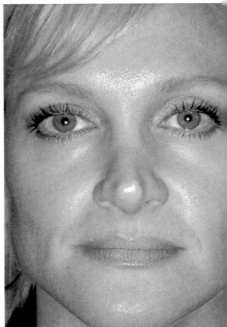

Figure 30: Before and After
BOTOX® Browlift

It is also possible to lift eyebrows
non-surgically with the customized use
of BOTOX® Cosmetic. I like to use
BOTOX® Cosmetic to not only improve
facial wrinkles and frown lines, but also
to perform beneficial facial re-balancing.
The photo you saw earlier was actually
an example of my BOTOX® Brow Lift
in Figure 30.

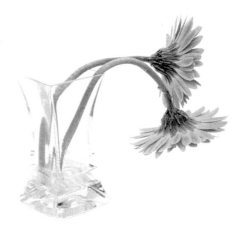

Festoons

Finally, festoons are a condition that many people believe are just an unfortunate part of aging. In fact, they commonly occur when the skin around the eyes and cheeks lose elasticity due to sun damage and stress forces in the underlying muscles. The skin of the lower eyelid becomes damaged, resulting in puffiness and severe drooping on the cheekbones below the eyelids.

Festoons are often misdiagnosed and, as a result, improperly treated or not treated at all. In extreme cases they can lead to peripheral vision loss, but even an average case can greatly impact the quality of a person's life.

It's safe to say that this is one of the most difficult eyelid conditions for cosmetic surgeons to correct. The most common options for treating festoons have included:

- Extensive incisional procedures with less-than-optimal results
- Direct excision of the festoons, resulting in very visible scars
- Medical therapy with marginal results

Individuals with festoons require additional treatment beyond normal blepharoplasty. In fact, a lower eyelid blepharoplasty or face lift can actually make the condition look worse and more noticeable. This is because removing the fullness of the lower eyelid above the festoon highlights the problematic area, making it even more obvious.

I am pleased to have refined and enhanced an effective, quick and much less invasive procedure method for correcting festoons. It provides my clients with great, natural-looking results. My revolutionary method was published in a medical textbook for cosmetic surgeons (*Master Techniques in Blepharoplasty and Periorbital Rejuvenation*[6]*)* and has been featured on television shows including *The Doctor Oz Show* and *The Doctors*. It takes advantage of the latest advances in laser application and wound healing to dramatically improve this difficult eyelid condition.

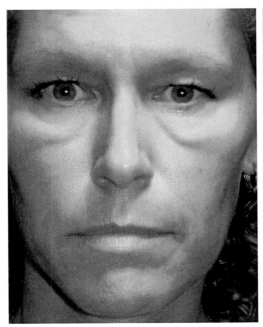 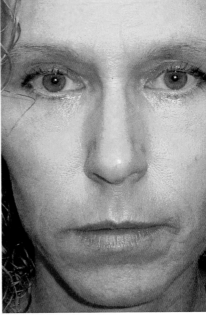

Figure 31: Before and After Laser Festoon RESET Treatment

Malar Mounds / Eyelid Festoons: Is There a "Natural" Remedy?

Patients often ask if there is a non-medical, "natural" remedy for malar bags and eyelid Festoons.

Non-surgically speaking, there is a "natural" remedy available, but it does not actually improve malar bags and eyelid Festoons; at most it can help prevent them from getting worse. This natural remedy is the regular use of sunblock and other sun protection. Wearing sunblock on all parts of your body exposed to sun on a daily basis prevents further sun damage to the skin and in turn prevents worsening of lower eyelid Festoons and Malar Mounds.

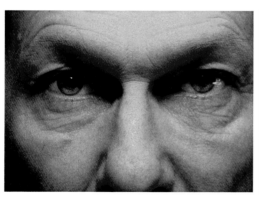 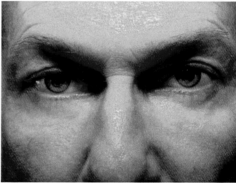

Figure 32: Patients often ask if there is a non-medical, "natural" remedy for malar bags and eyelid Festoons

Figures 33–35: Before and after Laser RESET
treatment for eyelid festoons

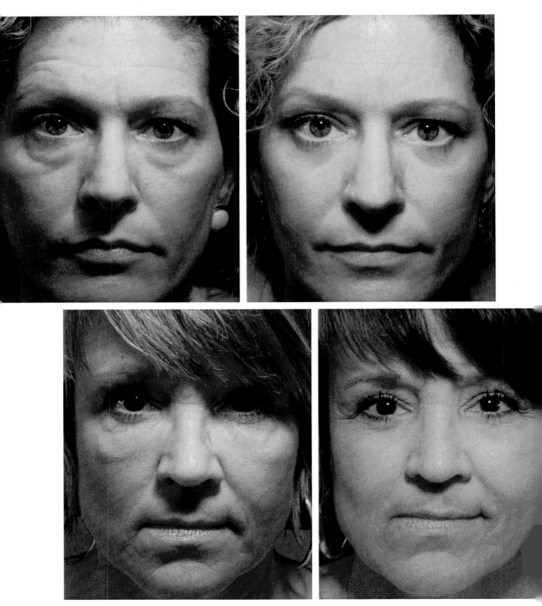

Another medical non-surgical way to somewhat reduce
Malar Mounds and eyelid Festoons involves the use of
medical products to improve the skin. One such product
is Tretinoin (commonly known as Retin-A), which
has been proven to help create new collagen in the skin.
Retin-A was discovered by Dr. Albert Kligman, who
was in the Dermatology Department at the medical
school where I trained, The University of Pennsylvania

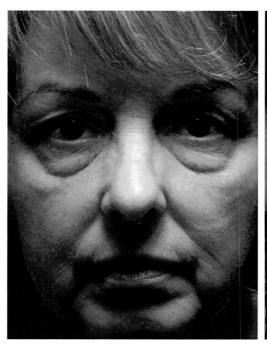 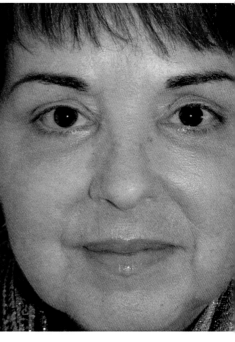

School of Medicine. Using Retin-A for many years
can improve the collagen and elastin levels in the skin,
which can help correct a main cause of many Malar
Mounds and Festoons—namely, damage to the skin over
time from the sun. That said, it is still not as effective
as surgical treatment options.

TRANSFORMATION

Another way that I help patients Restore, Reveal and Reclaim™ their natural beauty is through transformation.

Transformation involves helping patients reveal or uncover the beauty that has always been theirs, though they may not have known it or been able to see it. Unlike rejuvenation, which brings a patient's appearance back to a previous state, transformation can bring out a new balance, openness and symmetry.

Transformation can include:

• Certain eyelid and eyebrow elevation procedures

• Improving the line of a patient's nose through procedures like my 5-Minute Nose Job™

• Reducing heaviness above the eyelids which patients have had since birth

In these cases I am not reversing the effects of aging but rather helping patients improve and enhance features they've always had and that have always made them unhappy. It takes a special eye to see that which is possible in a person's face.

Transformation can bring about a very powerful change for patients in terms of the way they see themselves and the way the world sees them. For a glimpse at the way both transformation and rejuvenation have had incredible effects on some of my patients, take a look at the stories in the next chapter.

06

Natural Beauty in Action: Real Stories from Everyday People

We've all seen the good, the bad and the ugly of cosmetic procedures, but we rarely hear about the everyday people who've enhanced their appearance and non-verbal communication through properly customized cosmetic procedures. While these success stories may not make national news, they remain powerful and inspiring.

There may be people in your own life who've had this type of procedure without you even knowing it. That's what's so amazing about approaching cosmetic procedures with an eye to achieving enhanced natural beauty. People will know something is different and better about your appearance, but they won't be able to quite put their fingers on it.

My patients will often report that people have asked them:

Did you do something new with your hair?

Did you just come back from a day at the spa?

Have you lost weight?

DID YOU DO SOMETHING
NEW WITH YOUR
HAIR?

HAIR?

(...NO)

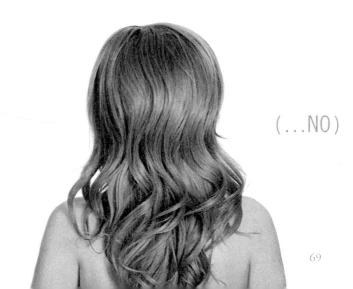

People will recognize that a person who's undergone a cosmetic procedure looks great, but they never guess why because the new look is so subtle, yet powerful.

Most patients don't want to walk away from a procedure with obvious signs that they've had work done — they just want to look like they did at a younger age. They want to regain some confidence in their appearance. They want to quit hearing, "Oh you look tired!" and, "Do you feel okay? You don't look so well." They want to improve the non-verbal cues they're sending out so that they can relate to the world more effectively.

When facial features are in balance, people respond to you differently. There are two reasons for this:

1 Because you feel better about yourself, and people are drawn to positive, well-balanced personalities

2 Because your non-verbal signals have been essentially cleaned up and optimized to match the true emotions and thoughts underneath

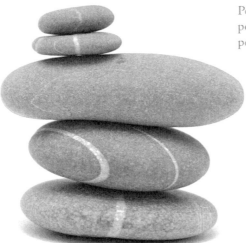

People are drawn to positive, well-balanced personalities

This is where I gain the most satisfaction in my work as a cosmetic surgeon. To see procedures rejuvenate and transform not only the physical appearance, but also the emotional well-being of my patients is so rewarding. So much emotion is tied up in our appearance, and improving the way someone looks can truly change their lives.

Whether you're dealing with drooping eyelids, deterioration of the facial tissue, or the puffy skin on the cheekbone known as festoons, there are treatments available to specifically target these areas. In my practice I take a customized approach to each client, first gaining an understanding of the look they desire and then merging their expectations with my Perfect Proportion Protocol based on the Golden Ratio, as covered in Chapter 4.

FREE FROM NEGATIVE NON-VERBAL MESSAGES

I'd like to share some of my own patients' stories to show you how cosmetic procedures aren't just for people in the Hollywood spotlight or those obsessed with physical perfection.

They're for everyday people who are on a journey to enhance their natural beauty. They're for people who want their non-verbal communication to match the way that they feel inside. They're for people who are beginning to understand that the new definition of true, natural beauty offers them hope—hope that they can achieve a well-balanced facial appearance and be free from the unwanted, negative non-verbal messages caused by unbalanced features.

FESTOON TREATMENT TRANSFORMS TWO WOMEN'S APPEARANCES

Donna was a 45-year-old patient whose under-eye bags made her "feel and look so much older than she really was." I had the pleasure of sharing her story, and my treatment of her, with Dr. Mehmet Oz on *The Dr. Oz Show* in a segment called "The Fix."

In addition to being told how tired she looked, Donna even had people asking her if she'd checked with her doctor about a sinus infection due to the severity of the puffiness under her eyes and on her cheekbones. She tried everything—from concealer to antihistamines to putting cucumbers and tea bags over her eyes—all to no avail. As her eye bags got worse she became more and more frustrated with the reflection she was seeing in the mirror. She wanted "to show the world who she really was," so she came to me for help.

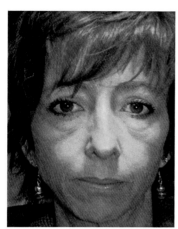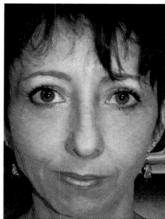

Figure 36: A transformation so extreme that even Dr. Oz himself was "flabbergasted"

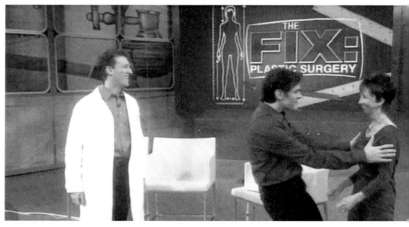

It was clear to me that what Donna was suffering from were festoons. Using my revolutionary laser treatment method, Donna's festoons were dramatically improved and she looked years younger and more refreshed. The transformation was so extreme that even Dr. Oz was "flabbergasted."

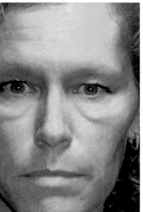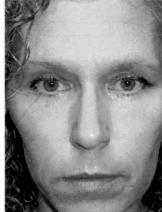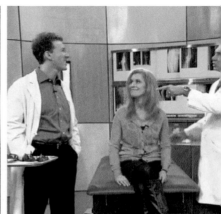

Figure 37: Erin had no idea that
her condition was more than
just normal under-eye bags

Erin was another woman suffering from festoons who
had tried everything she could think of to reduce the
baggy puffiness under her eyes. She had gone to three
plastic surgeons unsuccessfully, until she found herself
on the phone with her mother in tears over the hope-
lessness of her situation. I discussed Erin's story and
treatment on the television show *The Doctors*.

As with Donna, Erin had no idea that her condition
was more than just normal under-eye bags. By properly
diagnosing her festoons and using my laser treatment
to address them, I was able to dramatically improve the
bags under her eyes and on her cheekbones, leaving her
looking years younger. Her outside appearance finally
matched the beautiful spirit she had on the inside.

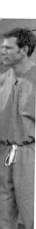

The extra good news is that as long as both women properly protect themselves from sun exposure, their skin will remain tight and smooth for many years, with no additional procedures needed.

SMALL BUSINESS OWNER RE-ENERGIZES HIS APPEARANCE

The patient in Figure 38 owned his own small business and was constantly hearing from customers that he looked tired and should get more rest. He felt fine but was concerned about the effect his appearance would have on getting new business. In addition, he was single and wanted to convey a more vibrant image to women he might meet. He took to wearing glasses in order to hide his eyelids from people, but this didn't feel comfortable to him and still didn't fully camouflage his tired-looking eyes from the world.

I helped him with my laser eyelid rejuvenation procedure, and the results were striking:

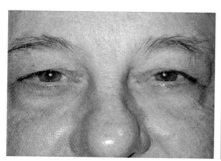
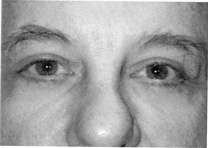

Figure 38: He was concerned about the effect his appearance would have on getting new business

Afterward he told me that other people were now relating to him better and that he had (thankfully!) stopped hearing comments about how tired he looked. In fact, though people didn't know what had happened to him they kept saying, "You look so healthy **and vibrant!** What have you been doing?"

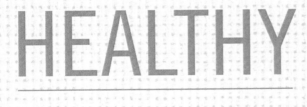

He simply smiled, keeping his secret to himself but knowing that his appearance was finally in line with the energy he felt inside.

HEALTHY

+

VIBRANT

ASIAN PATIENT MAINTAINS HER ETHNIC "LOOK" IN A NEW, REFRESHED WAY

In certain ethnic types such as Asian patients, redundant tissue can result in the presence of a "double eyelid." Procedures on these patients require special care to perform.

The patient below was tired of always looking tired. She'd always had a beautiful appearance, but over time she'd became frustrated with the heaviness above and puffiness below her eyes.

I had previously performed eyelid surgery on her niece and she had liked that I had improved her niece's appearance while still maintaining the natural Asian look of her eyelids. This was important to her — she didn't want to look "Western" or "Caucasian." She just wanted to look like a better, more refreshed version of herself.

The patient's lids had bothered her for months before she gathered the courage to go ahead with surgery, but when she did her results were amazing — subtle in their appearance yet powerful in their effect.

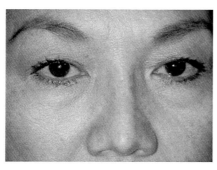 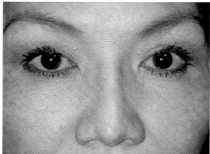

Figure 39: The patient above was tired of always looking tired

People told her she looked refreshed and energetic but they couldn't put their fingers on why. (It was her prerogative to keep the truth a secret from most people, although she did share it with some of her closest friends.)

SISTERS EXPERIENCE THEIR FIRST COSMETIC TREATMENT TOGETHER

A pair of sisters who were new to cosmetic treatments came to me and were quite nervous about having anything done.

I evaluated each woman and recommended my customized BOTOX® treatments as a starting procedure. They were ready to have the treatment right away — in fact, one sister actually gifted the other her BOTOX® treatment that same day!

I thought it was very sweet of her to treat her sister, and it was touching that they had came together to support one other. They made sure to ask questions about their treatments, such as whether their home environment would interfere with their treatment. (They lived out on a farm with animals around, and were concerned the environment might adversely affect their treatment outcome. I assured them it would not.)

The sisters came back a few weeks later, thrilled with the results from their customized BOTOX® treatments and asking what else I could recommend that didn't involve surgery. I suggested the volume replacement part of my Radiant*Lift*® procedure. Each had this treatment, and once again one sister covered the costs of the other's procedure. Their enthusiasm and camaraderie left a real impact on me.

When they returned to my office a few weeks later, they confided to me that their husbands wondered why they kept leaving the farm and coming into town. Their husbands had no idea they were having treatments! I was careful to leave both women with minimal signs that they had undergone treatments (except for the great, natural results).

It was touching that they
came together to support
each other

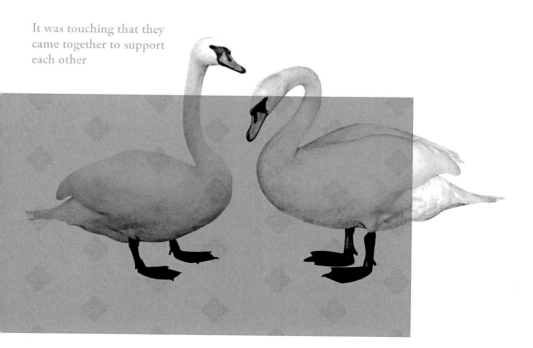

One sister shared that her relationship with her husband had become routine after many years. However, after the customized BOTOX® and Radiant*Lift*® procedures, her husband had started doing things for her like opening doors for her and taking her out on dates.

Of course, he didn't know she had undergone any procedures, but I believe he was reacting to the improved non-verbal messages she was now sending out as a result of those procedures.

The role my work had in bringing them closer together (with each other and with their husbands) really reinforced why I love doing what I do.

5-MINUTE NOSE JOB™ BRINGS THE OFFICE STAFF TO TEARS

One of my fondest memories is that of a patient I treated with my 5-Minute Nose Job™ procedure. The patient was around 60 years old and had told me that her nose had always bothered her, but that she'd lived with it because she wasn't enthusiastic about surgery and knew of no other options. When she learned about my 5-Minute Nose Job,™ she decided to give it a try.

When I finished her treatment, I handed her a mirror
so she could see the results for herself.

As she held the mirror and studied her new appearance,
tears slowly started rolling down her face. My staff and
I couldn't help but feel teary-eyed ourselves. I had just
helped fix a problem that had bothered this woman all
her life. It was a wonderful moment for me, for my staff
and for the patient. Check out these amazing results
in Figure 40.

5 MINUTES

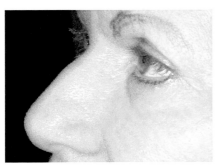
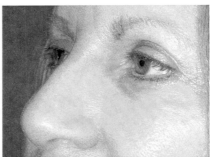

Figure 40: I had just helped fix
a problem that had bothered
this woman all her life

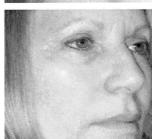
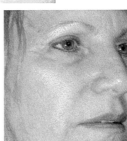

I truly love helping people because of stories like this one. It's amazing to think that my procedures can have such a strong impact on my patients, but I see it every day.

CUSTOMIZED BOTOX® TREATMENT TAKES YEARS OFF ONE CLIENT

"Amy" (not her real name) was a patient who had been coming to me for my customized BOTOX® treatments for a few years. In between two of her appointments I had begun to consider a new way to use BOTOX® to help bring out her natural beauty, and when she came in for her next treatment I suggested it to her. She allowed me to perform a more comprehensive custom BOTOX® treatment than I had previously done.

Two weeks went by and I ran into Amy at my kids' school play. The seats were full so I could only see the back of her head, but at the end of the play I made my way over to say hello and was stopped in my tracks. She looked amazing!

This treatment really helped bring out her natural beauty. Just see for yourself:

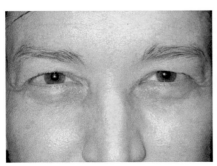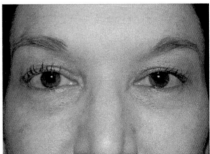

Amy shared with me that she'd recently visited a restaurant that she frequented regularly. The employee that served her had known her for a long time, and they'd often chatted about their lives. In talking with this person, Amy happened to mention that she was 46 years old.

The restaurant employee stopped, stared at Amy in shock and said, "I would have never guessed that you were in your 40s!" For the rest of the conversation, the employee kept saying, "I had no idea…I had no idea…"

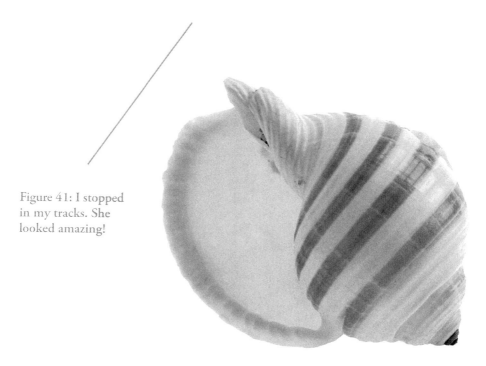

Figure 41: I stopped in my tracks. She looked amazing!

Amy told me that it had been a long time since she'd heard a compliment like that, and it had made her feel wonderful. She'd always been the youngest in her grade and had looked young for most of her life, but for the last decade or so she'd begun looking her actual age. As with many of my patients she'd become tired of people telling her she looked tired. She told me that now when people asked how she was doing, if she said she was feeling tired people responded by telling her that though she may feel tired, she looked great! What a wonderful reversal of responses!

If you've been living with an appearance that has been sending the wrong signals, or an appearance that you've secretly been unhappy with for years, these stories show that there is hope. You just need to find the right cosmetic surgeon to help you bring out the natural beauty that you have and deserve to show to the world. Check out the next chapter for some very important tips on how to do this.

People told her that she may feel tired, but she looks great!

THERE IS

HOPE

AS THESE
STORIES SHOW

07

11 Important Things Patients Should Know About Injectable Filler Treatments

Injectable fillers have become a large part of many cosmetic practices in the United States. This has been driven both by their ease of use and the impact they can have on reversing the signs of facial aging.

In a skilled hand, these products can lead to dramatic results for patients. In less skilled hands, they can lead to less dramatic results, facial distortion, and even scarring.

TYPES OF INJECTABLE FILLERS

There are a number of different types of injectable fillers, and more are coming onto the market every year.

There are currently three classes of fillers.

The first class is temporary fillers such as hyaluronic acids and collagen. Most of the temporary fillers currently used in the U.S. are hyaluronic acids such as Restylane®, Juvederm®, and Belotero®. These are nice to use not only because they give good results, but also because if necessary they can be reversed with an enzyme called Hyaluronidase.

The second class of fillers is the semi-permanent fillers such as Radiesse® and Sculptra®. These last longer but cannot be reversed when injected.

The final class is permanent fillers such as Bellafill and silicone. As their class name indicates, these also cannot be reversed once injected.

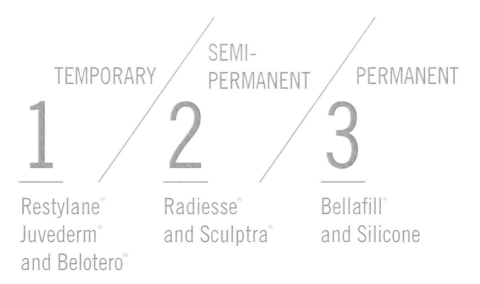

TEMPORARY

1

Restylane®
Juvederm®
and Belotero®

SEMI-
PERMANENT

2

Radiesse®
and Sculptra®

PERMANENT

3

Bellafill®
and Silicone

HOW CAN PATIENTS KNOW THEY'RE GETTING TREATMENTS THAT LEAD TO GOOD RESULTS?

Here are 11 key things to keep in mind when considering any type of injectable filler treatment:

1 FIND A QUALIFIED INJECTOR

First, it's important to find a qualified injector. It's best if this person is a doctor with a background in facial surgery, and it's even better if they have many years' experience using injectable fillers for facial rejuvenation themselves. (Some doctors have their staff do all of their injectable filler treatments.) I recommend that you evaluate the actual before-and-after photos of patients treated by the injector before you consider treatment with them.

2 THERE ARE NON-PHYSICIAN INJECTORS

There are non-physician injectors such as physician assistants and nurse practitioners who can be good, but it's important that they have many years' experience using fillers. Examine their before-and-after photos before considering treatment with them.

3

HYALURONIDASE AND NITROPASTE

The practitioner doing filler treatments must have Hyaluronidase and Nitropaste in their office. If they don't, then walk away. On rare occasions, fillers can cause complications such as an obstruction of blood flow to part of the face. This can lead to devastating results.

If the practitioner has Hyaluronidase and Nitropaste in their office they can be administered quickly to treat such problems. Once again, if an injector doesn't have these products in their office, walk away!

4

SEMI-PERMANENT AND PERMANENT FILLERS

Be careful with the use of semi-permanent and permanent fillers because they don't have the ability to be reversed. Still, they can be used very safely and effectively by practitioners who have years of experience in using them.

5 KNOW THE BACKGROUND OF THE PERSON INJECTING YOU

Know the background of the person injecting you. Does your injector have a background in facial procedures or are they a practitioner who decided to enter this field later in their careers? Today, injectable fillers are being provided by internal medicine doctors, dentists, ER doctors, pediatricians, OB-GYNs, nurses and physician assistants who may have little experience in facial anatomy.

Some can be good injectors, but only after extensive training and years of experience.

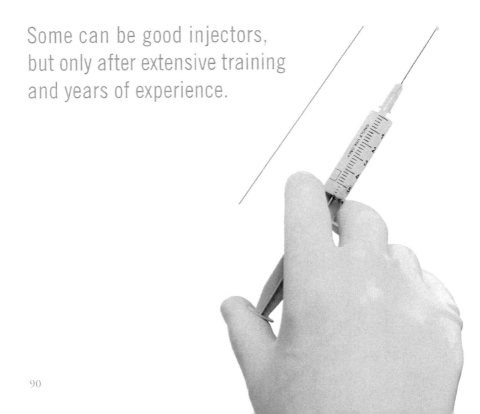

6 LOUPES

Experienced injectors often use magnifiers called loupes when injecting to enable them to better see the anatomy and avoid vessels. Ask if your injector uses these magnifiers. If they do, it usually means they're more careful and detail-oriented about their injectable procedures.

7 FILLER PLACEMENT UNDER THE EYES

It's important to be very careful with those practitioners who recommend injectable filler placement under the eyes. This often leads to more problems than it does successful outcomes.

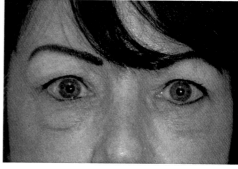

Figure 43: Bad result for fillers placed under the eyes

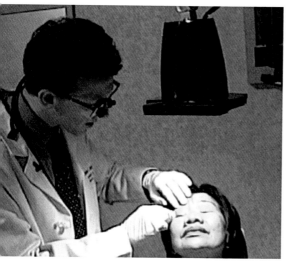

Figure 42: Ask if your injector uses these magnifiers

8

ANESTHESIA OPTIONS

Ask about the type of anesthesia options the practitioner offers. Options include topical anesthesia placed directly on the skin, injectable anesthesia and nerve block injected into the skin, and ice anesthesia.

Topical anesthesia combined with the anesthesia often incorporated into injectable fillers (e.g. Restylane® and Juvederm® often come with anesthesia mixed into them) is one option which can be good for injections in the cheeks to address lines that come from the nose down to the corner of the mouth (nasolabial folds) and for the lines that come from the corner of the mouth to the jaw line (melolabial folds). These products are appropriate for injections into the lip, but if the anesthesia used is only topical, expect to feel significant pain in the lips during the procedure.

Nerve blocks and direct injection of anesthesia usually provide the best comfort out off all of these options, making lips more comfortable during the injection process.

Ice is mildly effective and one of the least-sophisticated methods of reducing pain from injections.

Experienced injectors know how to offer all of these types of anesthesia. If the injector only offers topical anesthesia or ice, it usually means they don't have as much experience or skill in using injectable fillers.

9 LIP INJECTIONS

Only seek lip injections from very experienced injectors who have plenty of before-and-after photos to show you. The injection process is very artistic, and many injectors don't have a good artistic sense—many think they are just filling a line. Avoid these types of injectors.

10 FACIAL BALANCE

The best injectors know about and employ facial balance in the injection process. The practitioner needs to have exquisite knowledge of proper facial ratios and balance if they are going to be injecting a patient's face.

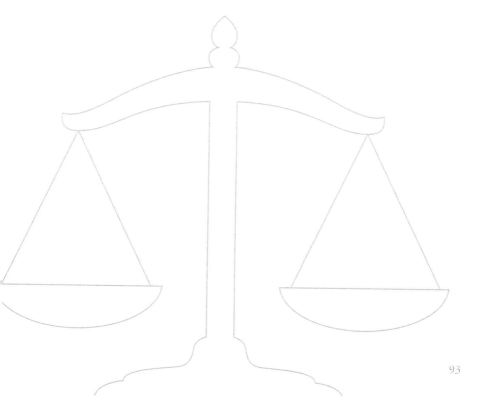

11

STOP USING ANY BLOOD THINNERS BEFORE THE PROCEDURE

Finally, it's important to stop using any and all blood thinners before the procedure, as they can increase the bruising you may see afterwards. These blood thinners aren't only medicines but include aspirin, headache powders with aspirin, gingko biloba, energy drinks, herbal teas, garlic, and ginseng among others. Avoid these for two weeks before the injection procedure and you'll have less bruising afterwards.

The bottom line? Injectable filler treatments are a safe and effective way of helping people restore their appearance to a more youthful and vibrant state. Following these 11 steps will make it more likely that you will receive a result that looks both beautiful and natural.

10 Tips for Choosing the Right Cosmetic Surgeon

People looking to have cosmetic surgery or a cosmetic procedure done often don't know the right questions to ask to ensure they'll get the care and results they desire. We tend to inherently trust doctors, but there are times when it's necessary to dig a little deeper and ask important questions to make sure your doctor's approach lines up with your expectations.

Here are 10 insider's tips to determine whether the surgeon you're considering is the right one for you:

1 LOOK FOR SPECIALIZATION.

Because the demand for cosmetic procedures is high, more doctors are joining the industry than ever before, but many lack the necessary specialization to perform specific procedures successfully. Thoroughly research your doctor to make sure that he or she has the experience necessary. Seek out "super-specialists" (doctors who exclusively practice cosmetic surgery in certain areas) as they are highly skilled in these areas and most likely to be on top of the latest medical advancements.

2 DON'T BE AFRAID TO ASK QUESTIONS.

It's your face and your life, so whether you need to know more about the procedure, the doctor's track record or recovery times, no question is too small or too "silly" to ask. You will be living with your results for the rest of your life, so you owe it to yourself to feel confident and secure about all aspects of your procedure.

3 DON'T UNDERESTIMATE RAPPORT WITH YOUR COSMETIC SURGEON.

If there is a clash of personalities or your doctor doesn't seem attentive to your questions and concerns during the initial consultation, it's best to keep looking. Communication and making sure you're on the same level are the keys to your doctor being able to bring about the results you envision.

4

DISCUSSING RISKS IS IMPORTANT

Beware of any doctor who dismisses the risks associated with surgery or who is unwilling to discuss potential complications. Your doctor should cover all of the possibilities and recovery scenarios so that you know what to expect and can fully understand the risks involved. Any doctor who downplays risks or is unwilling to discuss complications with you is a doctor you should not trust.

5

THINK OF THE INITIAL CONSULTATION AS AN INTERVIEW.

You are literally interviewing the doctor before giving them the right to take your appearance into his or her hands. Be sure you vet your surgeon as you would any potential job candidate. Inquire about fellowship training and specialized training for specific procedures, as well as the number of cases like yours that he or she has treated. Get a feel for your surgeon's philosophy and see if your visions mesh. There are many doctors out there from which to choose. Don't settle for someone with whom you're not 100% comfortable.

6

FOLLOW UP THE CONSULTATION WITH A THOROUGH BACKGROUND CHECK.

Verify the doctor's education, certification, and licenses through the medical board for the state in which he or she practices.

7 FEELING PRESSURED OR "SOLD TO" IS A RED FLAG.

A consultation should not be about pushing a doctor's services; it should be about your needs and questions. If your doctor makes you feel pressured, or is more interested in selling services than in hearing your vision for your treatment, keep looking.

8 CAREFULLY REVIEW "BEFORE-AND-AFTER" PHOTOS.

Examining the results of previous procedures can help you determine whether a doctor's work matches with your ultimate goals for your procedure.

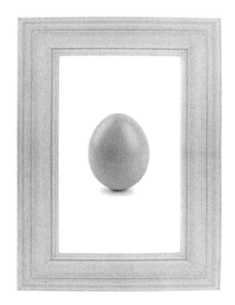

Determine whether a doctor's work matches with your ultimate goals

If you want a natural appearance and the after photos look glaring or lack facial balance, that's a sign to find a different doctor.

9 TAKE INTO CONSIDERATION THE AMBIANCE OF THE DOCTOR'S FACILITY AS WELL AS THE HELPFULNESS OF THE STAFF.

How you feel in the facility and how you are treated are important factors in your cosmetic procedure experience. The more comfortable and at ease you feel, the easier the procedure and recovery will be for you. As we've discussed, cosmetic procedures are not just physical procedures; they also involves complex emotional, mental and spiritual aspects. Knowing that you are in caring hands is key to making your experience the easiest it can be.

10 BEAR IN MIND THAT SURGERY ISN'T ALWAYS THE ANSWER.

As we've discussed, there are many non-surgical procedures and treatments that can help you to achieve your desired look for less cost and less recovery time. Ask your doctor to explain why he or she thinks a particular procedure is right for your situation and whether there is another, less-invasive route that could provide similar results.

09

10 Common Questions Patients Ask About Cosmetic Treatments and Surgeries

Over the years I've often heard the same questions and concerns from patients, and chances are that you have some of these same questions yourself. Here are the 10 questions I most commonly hear in my practice.

1

WHAT KIND OF HEALING PROCESS IS INVOLVED IN COSMETIC PROCEDURES?

There are multiple levels of healing depending upon which procedure you are having done.

In some minimal-impact procedures such as non-invasive laser or light treatments or BOTOX® treatments, it takes mere hours for some of the transient pinkness to fade away.

The next level of healing is necessary when injections are made more deeply in the skin such as in my Radiant*Lift*® procedure. With procedures like this, swelling and some bruising can occur. If there is bruising it can be covered with makeup after one day and usually resolves on its own over the course of the next two weeks.

The final level of healing occurs when incisions are made through the skin or when levels of the skin are treated to allow new skin to come through. In these cases there is initial inflammation of the wound and then new collagen and elastic fiber growth. An initial 1–2 weeks of recovery are often required before one feels comfortable going out and about with makeup on. Full resolution of swelling can take months, and final healing from these deeper procedures often takes about a year. But it is worth it; the results for most of these procedures are like a "reset" button that gives you new, beautiful, healthier skin and/or a new you!

The level of healing depends
upon which procedure you
are heaving done

2 IS IT SELFISH OR NARCISSISTIC TO WANT COSMETIC PROCEDURES?

Absolutely not. Why do people wear makeup or even comb their hair? It's because we're inherently social beings and we all want to be able to connect with others as easily as possible. This includes taking care of our appearances so that they communicate what we want them to about us. There is nothing selfish or narcissistic about wanting your non-verbal messages to match the way you feel inside.

I consider myself a communication facilitator: I help clean up the aberrant messages my patients' faces are sending; I bring their appearances into better balance with their internal states.

I'm passionate about helping people Restore, Reveal and Reclaim® their natural beauty and, in doing so, optimizing their non-verbal messages so that the world relates to them in a better way.

3

HOW DO I KNOW I HAVE THE RIGHT COSMETIC SURGEON?

New doctors enter the cosmetic surgery field every day, and it's hard to do everything well. While there are some great surgeons who are able to work successfully on a wide range of procedures, most of the best surgeons specialize in a specific area.

Finding specialists with good training, years of experience in their field and a history of performing procedures of the type you're considering is a good place to start. Your surgeon should be board-certified and specialty- or fellowship-trained in the treatment area you're interested in. They should use accredited facilities for their procedures and be licensed by the state in which they operate. They should also regularly keep up with advances in their field by attending specialty meetings, reading medical journals and attending seminars and lectures.

It's very important to interview your surgeon in person, as you should feel comfortable with them and they with you. A good surgeon will take the time to fully examine and educate a prospective patient about the procedures they recommend. If a doctor is rushing through their initial meeting with you, you should wonder if they will be very patient and caring for you after you've gone through a procedure with them.

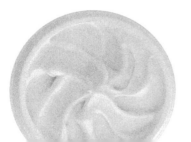

It's important that you
have a good connection with
your surgeon

Finally, it's important that you have a good connection with your surgeon, because the relationship between a cosmetic surgeon and his or her patient is a crucial and intimate one that depends on rapport and trust between both parties.

Check out Chapter 8 for some basic tips to keep in mind when choosing a cosmetic surgeon.

4 WILL IT BE OBVIOUS TO OTHERS THAT I'VE HAD WORK DONE?

To answer this I'd like you to first consider the example of a patient who wants to reduce the lines on their forehead. An unsophisticated doctor may treat these lines directly with a procedure like BOTOX® but it's important to dig deeper and ask why a person has these lines. Often it's because as we age and suffer sun damage our brows and eyelids fall, prompting the forehead to act as a compensatory muscle to help lift the brows and lids. Treating the symptoms of this (forehead lines) rather than the underlying cause can result in a weakening of their compensation, making the brows collapse into the eyelid space. Not only will it be clear that the person has had work done, but the results will be less than optimal.

I prefer instead to target the muscles that are pulling down the brow in the first place so that the brows raise more naturally. This results in less severe forehead lines as well as a more open and balanced appearance.

The best surgical results are powerful yet subtle. I want people to see my patients and know something about them has improved, but not be able to put their finger on exactly what has changed.

My patients often hear comments like, "Have you been working out?" "Have you lost weight?" "Your hair looks great!" "Are you wearing new earrings?" These people's subconscious minds perceive a positive change in my patients but are unable to process a conscious awareness of the source of that change. My patients can smile and say "Thank you" while keeping the truth a secret only they know.

Many people are afraid of results that don't look natural. Achieving natural results requires a sophisticated understanding of how our faces change with time and how to identify and treat the cause of certain problems, not just the effects of those problems. Paying attention to the natural ratios of the face also allows me to create powerful yet subtle results.

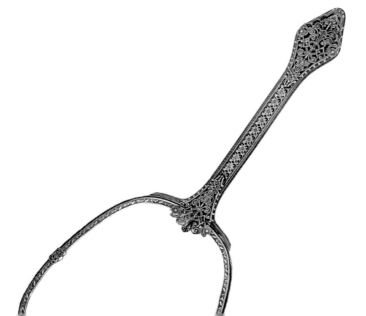

5

I DON'T HAVE TIME FOR A LONG PROCEDURE OR RECOVERY. WHAT ARE MY BEST OPTIONS?

Luckily, today there are many non-invasive ways to help patients which involve minimal downtime. Modern laser techniques can improve skin tone and balance through quick office procedures with minimal recovery periods.

Neuromodulators such as BOTOX® can help rejuvenate a face by improving the lift of the eyebrows and smoothing frown lines and crow's feet. Facial rebalancing can be done with my Radiant*Lift*® procedure, in which I correct volume loss in the face and improve skin tone and appearance. These are both quick office procedures.

New technologies and the artful use of facial volumizers can give patients great results without long recovery periods.

HAVE YOU

BEEN WORK-ING OUT?

(...NO)

WHAT IS INVOLVED IN A COSMETIC CONSULTATION?

Each surgeon's consultation will be slightly different, but there should be certain commonalities among them all.

In my office a consultation begins with the patient meeting my staff and being initially evaluated by my Cosmetic Technicians. Then they meet me and we talk about their specific concerns.

Next comes an evaluation process where I examine the patient's face, skin, facial balance, bone structure, eyelid region and eyes. If any procedure will involve the eye region it's important to examine the eye itself to ensure that it is healthy enough to undergo surgery in that area. For the same reason I also examine a patient's heart and lungs to make sure they are healthy enough for any proposed procedures.

I will then review my specific findings with the patient, and we will have an in-depth discussion of the treatment options that are available to them. I will give a full explanation of any procedures suggested so that the patient understands the pre-care process, the treatment process, the recovery process and the risks involved with the procedures. I will then present before-and-after photos of other patients who have had similar procedures.

Finally, we'll go over any remaining questions and answers, and then (depending on patient interest at that point), we'll discuss costs as well as possible dates available for the procedure(s).

7

HOW DO I KNOW IF I HAVE FESTOONS?

Our faces are highlighted by the light that surrounds us. Most of the time some form of light is shining down on us from above, whether it's the sun or overhead lights in a room. This light casts highlights and shadows over our faces that often spotlight festoons. It's a game of light and shadows that highlight certain convexities and concavities on our faces. As we age our faces lose certain convexities, and this makes us look older.

Festoons in specific are often most noticeable right after you wake up. They typically appear as swollen mounds on the cheeks which can be moved easily from side to side.

Light casts highlights and shadows over our faces that often spotlight festoons

Looking in a mirror with a light overhead is a good way to check to see if you have festoons, or Malar Mounds as they're also known. They often lie below the bags which form directly below the lower eyelid lashes. Festoons form further down the lower eyelid region and onto the cheek.

Thankfully, I have a treatment that helps both of these conditions and can have a dramatic effect on a patient's appearance and non-verbal communication.

8 WHAT ARE MY BEST OPTIONS IF I WANT A NATURAL APPEARANCE?

The key is to seek treatment from a physician who is highly skilled and well-versed in the natural ratios of the face. Only by respecting these ratios can you achieve results that are powerful, yet natural and subtle.

9 HOW CAN I BE SURE I'LL HAVE A POSITIVE OUTCOME FROM MY TREATMENT?

First, realistic goals and attitudes are critical for a patient. You should have surgery done for yourself, not to try to please another person. Although "perfection" isn't possible with even the best treatments, dramatic improvements are possible through the application of the Golden Ratio, as we have discussed.

A patient's age, skin type, general health, family background and especially prior sun exposure can all affect the eventual outcome of a treatment.

You should stop all medications and products that might cause bleeding before a treatment, as long as it is safe to do so. This should be checked with your primary care physician. This list includes products such as aspirin, fish oil, vitamin E supplements, gingko biloba, garlic, herbal teas, and supplements.

Ceasing smoking is also important as it increases the healing blood flow necessary for a quick recovery.

Following all of your surgeon's directions after a procedure is very important in order to ensure optimal results.

Finally, it's crucial to protect yourself from sun exposure with the daily application of a sun block that blocks both UVA and UVB rays.

As a specialist in facial rejuvenation, I'm often asked by patients what product they can use to keep themselves looking young. They typically ask about special creams, ointments, and serums. My answer to them is that the best thing people can do is simply to wear sunscreen daily; it's one of the best ways to keep a person looking young. Recent research from Australia supports this advice.[7]

Of all of the factors affecting the aging of our skin, the biggest is photo aging, or aging of the skin due to exposure to the sun. And the single best way to help prevent skin from this aging is through sun protection. It's been estimated that 90% of all wrinkles, age spots, and skin discoloration is due to sun or tanning bed exposure.

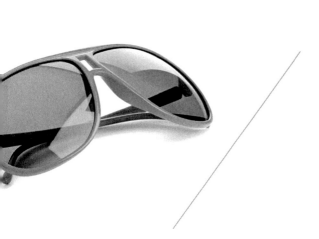

90%

It's been estimated that
90% of aging is due
to sun or tanning bed
exposure

THE ABCS OF UV

In order to properly protect ourselves against the sun,
it's important to understand exactly how it affects our
skin. When the sun shines down on the earth and
warms us, it contains a number of different types of
light rays. Visible light is the most obvious as it allows us
to see, but another type of light ray is invisible yet very
damaging to us. These are Ultraviolet (UV) rays, which
themselves can be broken down into several parts.

The first type of UV ray is UVA rays. UVA rays acceler-
ate skin aging. They have a long wavelength that allows
them to penetrate deeply into the skin, through the
epidermis and down into the dermis where they can
fracture collagen and elastic fibers. These rays are present
all day long, from sun up to sun down — they even
have the ability to penetrate clouds and car windows.

The next type is UVB rays. These cause redness in the skin and are responsible for sunburn. They are most prevalent from 10:00 a.m. to 4:00 p.m. and have a shorter wavelength that can't penetrate as deeply into the skin.

The last type is UVC rays. These are toxic to life and absorbed by the ozone layer.

SPF (the number you see on your sunscreen bottles) is an acronym for Sun Protection Factor. It primarily measures protection against UVB rays, but new guidelines are helping consumers understand whether products help against UVA rays as well. This is very important as it's critical for us to use sun protection products that block both UVA and UVB rays.

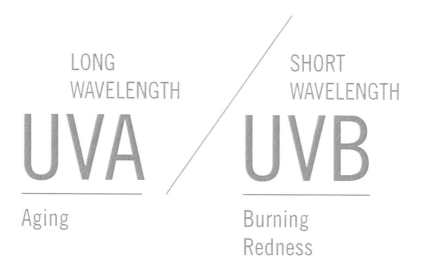

LONG
WAVELENGTH
UVA

Aging

SHORT
WAVELENGTH
UVB

Burning
Redness

Figure 34: It's critical for us to
use sun protection products that
block both UVA and UVB rays.

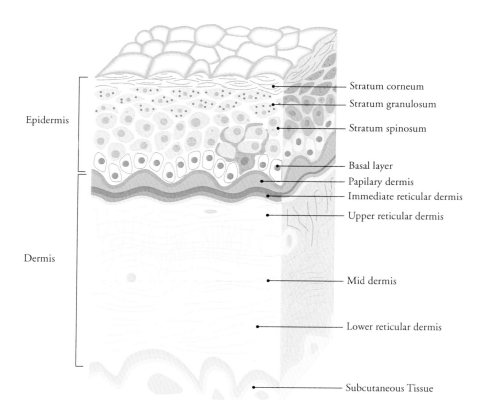

Epidermis

Dermis

Stratum corneum
Stratum granulosum
Stratum spinosum

Basal layer
Papilary dermis
Immediate reticular dermis
Upper reticular dermis

Mid dermis

Lower reticular dermis

Subcutaneous Tissue

We should not be protecting ourselves only on certain
occasions; incidental exposure matters! Every moment
that skin is exposed to the sun, radiation is creating
some damage. Skin damage from the sun doesn't just
occur when you're spending a day at the beach; it also
occurs when you're walking from your home to your
mailbox or driving your car.

To help protect our skin it is critical to wear sun protection every day, on all exposed areas. Sun damage is cumulative, and years of daily small sun damage can add up to a much older appearance and a greater amount of damage to skin.

Take a look at the examples of UV exposure over time in Figure 44.

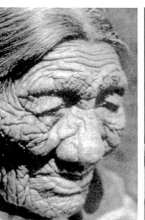 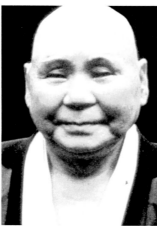

Figure 44: The woman on the left is only 58 years old. She worked in the sun most of her life, and her skin reflects this exposure.

The man on the right is 78 years old. He is a monk and spent most of his days inside meditating.

Notice the difference in the qualities of their skin. This is what happens with daily sun exposure over time.

The next example is equally striking. This person is a truck driver, and over his career one side of his face has always been facing the window where the sun would come through and warm his cheek. Remember how I mentioned that UVA rays can penetrate car windows?

After years of driving a truck, the two sides of this man's face have visibly different levels of skin aging as a result of his UVA exposure over time:

One side of his face has always been facing the window

Using computers we can superimpose the left and right sides of his face and create the following two examples. The first picture is what this man would look like if both sides of his face matched the less exposed skin on his right side.

The next is what he would look like if his entire face had the more exposed skin currently on his left side.

Notice the big difference in how we perceive his age between these two pictures. Sun exposure really matters!

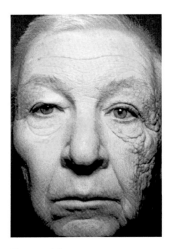
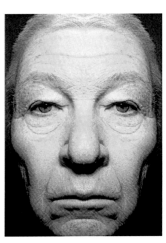
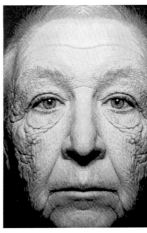

Figure 45:
Original image

Right side
mirrored

Left side
mirrored

WHAT THE AUSTRALIA STUDY MEANS

The research I mentioned earlier, which was done at the Queensland Institute of Medical Research and published in the journal Annals of Internal Medicine, studied 900 men and women over the course of four years. One group used regular sunscreen daily and the other used it only occasionally. As I have been suggesting for years, those who used it daily experienced 24% less skin aging than those who only used it sporadically.

These results have more significance than simply preventing skin aging. The same sun exposure that ages our skin also contributes to skin cancers. Protecting our skin from the sun doesn't just help us look younger — it also helps us stay healthier by reducing our chances of skin cancer.

I have many ways that I can reverse sun damage using my laser skin resurfacing procedures (see below), but it's always best if we can prevent sun damage in the first place.

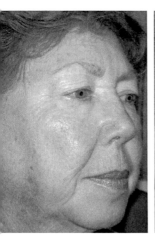 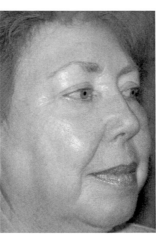

Figure 46: Protecting our skin from the sun doesn't just help us look younger; it also helps us stay healthier

10

ARE COSMETIC TREATMENTS SAFE?

Overall, yes. However, there are certain risks involved with any procedure. This goes back to your initial consultation with your physician and why rapport with them is so important.

Any and all risks involved in a potential treatment should be discussed during a consultation. A patient must also be sure to inform the surgeon about their specific medical history so that a true assessment of surgical risks can be ascertained.

Although risks are possible with any procedure, with proper preparation and post-procedure care, complications and problems are rare.

CONCLUSION

In spite of the bad rap they've gotten, cosmetic surgery and cosmetic procedures can actually do wonders in terms of enhancing patients' natural beauty in subtle yet powerful ways that can be transformational in their lives.

The key lies in recognizing that true beauty isn't a fad and isn't something that can be achieved by a nearsighted focus on one limited aspect of a patient's appearance. By following the Golden Ratio — a formula that has enabled us to recognize beauty for centuries — a cosmetic surgeon will be able to produce results that are balanced and natural-looking, and which enhance rather than distract from a patient's overall appearance.

It is important for patients to carefully investigate their cosmetic surgeon to make sure that he or she understands the nature of true beauty and is able to perform the specialized, customized procedure(s) that will help them rediscover their own natural beauty. Not every surgeon has this ability, so ensuring that you are in the hands of a specialist is key in getting the results you both desire and deserve.

So much of our lives are affected by our appearances. The way we are viewed by the world, the way we view ourselves, and the way we communicate with others are all influenced by the non-verbal cues we send out. When these cues are aligned with who we really are and how we truly feel inside, our relationships with others and our confidence in ourselves can be drastically improved.

I hope that our examination of the nature of true beauty has opened your eyes to the potential we all have to Restore, Reveal and Reclaim® our own unique beauty. If you have any questions or would like to discuss anything in this book further, please don't hesitate to contact me using the information below:

Adam J. Scheiner, M.D.
813.367.1915
www.adamscheinermd.com

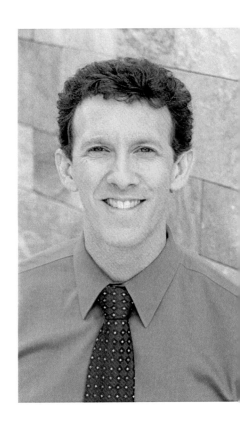

ACKNOWLEDGMENTS

I would like to thank and acknowledge the many people who have made this book a reality:

First and foremost, I wish to acknowledge my wonderful wife and family, who have allowed me the time needed to be a physician who is dedicated to the care of his patients.

Next, I'd like to thank my friend and advisor Elizabeth Kanna, who has inspired me and made it possible for me to help patients from around the world.

I'd like to thank my mentor and friend Sterling Baker, M.D., under whose tutelage I learned and was inspired to be a facial laser surgeon.

I'd like to thank my partners in my practice, who have supported me in my continued professional growth.

I'd like to thank my parents, who have always been supportive and inspirational in my life and who taught me to strive for excellence and be of service to others.

I'd like to thank Janet, who helped me reach a broader audience about my unique procedures and methodology.

I'd like to thank my staff—Toni, Sally, Judy, Ann, Bea, Leslie, Nancy and Kathi who are wonderful partners in the care of our patients.

Finally, I'd like to thank my patients, who continually move me and inspire me to become a better doctor and surgeon.

REFERENCES

1 Marquardt, Stephen. (2011, October 31). Marquardt Beauty Analysis. Retrieved from *http://www.beautyanalysis.com/*

2 Gorman, Carol Kinsey. (2011). *Silent Language of Leaders: How Body Language can Help — Or Hurt — How You Lead.* San Francisco, CA: Jossey-Bass (A Wiley Imprint).

3 Mehrabian, Albert. (1981). *Silent Messages: Implicit Communication of Emotions and Attitudes* (2nd ed.). Belmont, CA: Wadsworth.

4 Etcoff, Nancy. (2000). *Survival of the Prettiest: The Science of Beauty.* New York: Anchor Books (A Division of Random House, Inc.).

5 Russell Richard. (2009). *A sex difference in facial contrast and its exaggeration by cosmetics Perception.* Volume 38, pages 1211–1219

6 Massry, Guy G. MD, et al. (2011). *Master Techniques in Blepharoplasty and Periorbital Rejuvenation.* New York: Springer.

7 M.C.B. Hughes, G.M. Williams, P. Baker, and A.C. Green. (4 June 2013). "Sunscreen and Prevention of Skin Aging. A Randomized Trial." *Annals of Internal Medicine* (volume 158, pages 781-790).

Made in the USA
San Bernardino, CA
08 February 2018